KEEPING WELL

BRITTANY WISNIEWSKI

KEEPING WELL

An Anti-Cancer Guide to Remain in Remission

NEW YORK

LONDON • NASHVILLE • MELBOURNE • VANCOUVER

Keeping Well

An Anti-Cancer Guide to Remain in Remission

Published in New York, New York, by Morgan James Publishing in partnership with Difference Press. Morgan James is a trademark of Morgan James, LLC.
www.MorganJamesPublishing.com

ISBN 9781642799637 paperback
ISBN 9781642799644 eBook
ISBN 9781642799651 audiobook
Library of Congress Control Number: 2019957354

Cover Design Concept:
Nakita Duncan

Interior Design by:
Christopher Kirk
www.GFSstudio.com

Editor:
Cory Hott

Book Coaching:
The Author Incubator

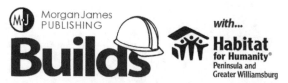

Morgan James is a proud partner of Habitat for Humanity Peninsula and Greater Williamsburg. Partners in building since 2006.

Get involved today! Visit
MorganJamesPublishing.com/giving-back

For my mom, Kathy Wisniewski, who passed away from stage four breast cancer when I was nineteen. She was the kindest soul and an angel on earth. She continues to guide me through my life and definitely through the writing of this book.

TABLE OF CONTENTS

Chapter 1:   I Am Choosing to Remain Cancer-Free. 1

Chapter 2:   I Am Open to Receive Guidance. 7

Chapter 3:   I Am Keeping My Body Well by Listening to
             What It Has to Say .13

Chapter 4:   I Understand How My Body Works,
             So I Know How to Heal It 17

Chapter 5:   I Know My Body Has the Ability to Heal
             Itself and I Assist It in Every Way 41

Chapter 6:   I Create A Healthy Environment
             All Around Me 47

Chapter 7:   I Welcome All Emotions to Be Healed 55

Chapter 8:   I Have A Clear Path to Success in
                 Keeping My Body Well 61

Chapter 9:   I Will Live My Life with Ease and Grace 69

Chapter 10: I Am Dedicated to Healing My Body
                 and Keeping Well Because I Am
                 Worthy of Having A Perfectly Healthy
                 Body and Feeling Great 75

Acknowledgments 79

Thank You 81

About the Author 83

Endnotes 0

Chapter 1:

I AM CHOOSING TO REMAIN CANCER-FREE

"It's not the big things that add up in the end; it's the hundreds, thousands, or millions of little things that separate the ordinary from the extraordinary."
– Darren Hardy

Each day you make hundreds of decisions that collectively affect the course of your life. Daily decisions made over the course of ten years can be life-altering. What if you ate one bowl of conventional, non-organic cereal every morning? It's not very convincing if I tell you that it could have a possible cancer-causing effect on the body, is it? When you accumulate one bowl of cereal over the course of ten years you get 3,650 bowls containing trace amounts of the cancer-causing pesticide glyphosate and maybe some yellow number 5 dye (which has already been banned in Europe for its correlation to colon cancer). This is the power of your daily choices.

If We Don't Program Ourselves, Our Environment Will

What were the earliest meals you learned how to cook? There's a good chance they were recipes that you learned from your parents, grandparents, or other family members, right? Our eating habits are developed early in life based on family traditions. Personally, my favorites were pasta salad, coffee, and pierogis (I'm Polish if you can't tell) – weird combination, I know. I got locked into being a coffee drinker very early on. My bushi (a terribly Americanized way of saying grandmother in Polish) would seriously brag about how she never drank a glass of water in her life, like it was something to be proud of. She had a cup of coffee and a piece of cake every single day. To this day, coffee remains my biggest vices. Thanks a lot, Bushi!

If I hadn't learned about diet and nutrition by doing my own research, I would have never changed the eating habits of my upbringing. This also goes for lifestyle changes other than diet. How have your physical activity, family stress, and even the commercial products you use, like cleaning supplies and body-care products, been influenced by your family or upbringing?

Most of the time it's not the cancer gene but the common risk factors they share that runs in families.

Pottenger's Cats

We do not start with a perfectly clean slate of health when we are born. We are the result of the generations before us. You know the generation that use to spray DDT (dichlorodiphenyltrichloroethane) on just about everything. DDT was one of the first man-made insecticides and is still to this day found in some breast milk samples. DDT stays in the environment for a long time and accumulates in fatty tissues of the body such as the breast. Breast milk is often used to measure a population's exposure.

In 2004, the Environmental Working Group (EWG) analyzed the umbilical cord blood of ten newborn babies in the U.S. and they found 287 industrial chemicals in the blood of all ten. Findings were a combination of common consumer product chemicals, waste byproducts, and chemicals that had already been banned in the United States prior to the child's birth. "This is the human 'body burden' – the pollution in people that permeates everyone in the world, including babies in the womb" (https://www.ewg.org/research/body-burden-pollution-newborns).

Among the first ah-ha moments for me when it comes to researching why so many people are getting cancer in this generation was learning about the Pottenger study. In the 1940s, Dr. Francis Marion Pottenger Jr. conducted a ten-year study on four generations of cats that correlated diet and disease. His experiment was to determine the effects of heat-processed food vs. raw meat and milk. Now, obviously cats naturally don't have a means of cooking their catch of the day, so only one of the diets in the study was natural and healthy for them.

All four generations of the cats that ate raw meat and milk remained healthy throughout their lives.

The first generation of the processed food – eating cats developed diseases and illness near the end of their lives. The second generation developed diseases and illness in the middle of their lives. The third generation developed diseases and illness in the beginning of their lives, and some even died at a very young age. There was no fourth generation because the third-generation parents were either sterile or the cats died in utero. It's simply evolution; nature does not allow the weak to procreate.

What generation of cats are we? Your toxic burden began when you were still in the womb. The body is like a bucket slowly filling with toxins from the past. When will it overflow and cause problems? Baby boomer parents, like mine, die from cancer toward the middle of their lives. Childhood cancer is higher than at any time in history. In 2018 the CDC reported that about ten percent of women had difficulty getting pregnant or staying pregnant. Weaknesses are genetically passed down in a slow decline until someone along the line makes a change. Are you going to change the course in a positive direction for yourself and those closest to you?

Women are directly responsible for the next two generations. Your grandmother carried a part of you when she was pregnant with your mother. A female fetus is born with all the eggs she will ever have in her lifetime. So you were a tiny, unfertilized egg in your grandmother's uterus – perhaps a raisin if your Bushi never had a glass of water in her life.

In all seriousness, how cool is that? Ladies, when you heal yourself, you are directly healing the next two generations to come.

What's It Worth To You?

You are ninety percent in control of this statement. Cancer is mostly a lifestyle and environmental disease caused by toxins, pollutants, smoking, diet, alcohol, sun exposure, infections, radiation, stress, obesity, and physical inactivity.* Genes get mutated from the influences of these various factors, not just from bad genetics. With only five to fifteen percent of cancers being caused by genetics, the remaining percentage is in your hands. This book is a guide to taking back that ninety percent.

*Cancer is often a preventable disease that requires major lifestyle changes.[1]

One of my favorite books is 'The Compound Effect' by Darren Hardy . It should be a required read in high schools, I'm telling you. I highly recommend it as your next read, but don't put this one down quite yet. If you're looking to change anything in your life, those small daily choices are vastly overlooked. You choose your destiny with these decisions. When you can make educated anti-cancer choices on a daily basis, that ninety percent is looking pretty bright.

I created the Keeping Well journey to set the foundation of healing for you and for those around you, as a means to healing your generation and those to come. My wish isn't just for you to remain in remission but to end the cycle of cancer for good.

"I've never seen any life transformation that didn't begin with the person in question finally getting tired of their own nonsense."

– Elizabeth Gilbert

Chapter 2

I AM OPEN TO RECEIVE GUIDANCE

"Life is tough, but so are you!"
- Unknown

I wrote this book as if I was writing it for my mom to read post–breast cancer treatments. My mom was diagnosed with stage two breast cancer when I was in elementary school. She did the recommended surgery, chemotherapy, and radiation and was deemed in remission for the next ten years. Exactly ten years later, she started getting chest pain and felt a lump in the middle of her chest. I still remember the day she told me that she had breast cancer for the second time. I had just graduated from high school and was in skincare school at the time. This time it was found in her sternum bone and had metastasized to a stage four "terminal" cancer. I put the word terminal purposely in quotation marks because I now know that stage four "terminal" cancer does not have to be a death sentence. I have met many medically deemed terminal cancer patients who are thriving today, many years after their diagnoses. The body's ability to heal when you have hope, change the environment in which you got sick, and give it the proper tools is truly amazing. Doctors call this spontaneous remission. It should be called "I put in the work, changed my unhealthy habits, and had faith in my body's ability to heal itself" remission. This book is a collection of the anti-cancer, detoxification, and self-healing practices I have discovered in the nine years since my mom passed away. In those nine years, I have grieved by tirelessly and passionately pursuing all of the knowledge I could on self-healing and preventing cancer.

Just a few months after my mom died, I started my journey working at an organic wellness center that focuses on body detoxification. I jumped right into learning everything I could and gained firsthand knowledge from working next to colon hydrotherapists. I studied colon health, became a regenerative detoxification specialist at the International School of Detoxification and got certified in plant-based nutrition from eCornell. I took countless courses in: herbalism, energy healing, Reiki, anatomy, and many more. I am currently a Traditional Naturopathy student at New Eden School of Natural Health. Through all of this, I was my own experiment. I have tried just about every detox in the book, every health fad, and every supplement, and I will continue to do so. I love to teach from personal experience, and I credit myself with not being biased toward just one way of healing. That is perhaps the greatest thing I have learned on this journey. One particular healing method does not serve all. This book is a guide for prevention through an anti-cancer lifestyle.

I have always had a passion for living healthfully and have known I would be doing something in the health and wellness field since I was a child; however, it wasn't until my mom died that the learning started. It all started with one DVD, a bread crumb left by my mom leading me toward my destiny. This DVD was *Crazy Sexy Cancer* by Kris Carr. If you're not familiar, it is all about Kris's cancer journey through learning about holistic and nutritional therapies after her cancer diagnosis. Through this journey, she stopped the progression of her cancer and now has a thriving wellness business. Watching this documentary left me a sobbing mess. My mom had died no more than one week before I watched this DVD that I had found in her room, and I was SO mad at myself. I was so mad that I had not watched this while she was alive. I also wondered if she had watched it herself. Either way, I most definitely knew she wasn't doing any natural therapies mentioned, which I was sure could have improved her quality of life at that time.

My mom was seemingly healthy prior to her diagnosis. She loved her workout VHS tapes, she had bran muffins for breakfast, and she made sure to drink plenty of water. She was one of the healthiest moms I knew in the early 2000's, so why did my seemingly healthy mom get cancer? She also tested negative for the BRCA gene. So, what went wrong enough for her to get breast cancer? Fast-forward to today, and I know health goes way deeper than bran muffins and adequate water intake, but also the common factor in her life at those two times when she got diagnosed was extreme stress. Stress increases cortisol in the body causing inflammation which reduces immune function and leaves you susceptible to disease. Stress also induces cancer metastasis.[*2]

I'm sure my mom wouldn't appreciate me telling you all of this, but for the sake of helping others, I don't think she would mind. Looking back and analyzing my mom's case from a holistic point of view, I want to first note the cancer-causing factors in her life at the time of her diagnosis.

- Extreme emotional life stressors prior to diagnosis
- Chronic constipation

- Standard American diet (meat, cheese, low-quality food, not enough nutritional value especially in vitamins and antioxidants, 100% non-organic diet)
- Cellular damage from past chemotherapy (chemotherapy is a cytotoxic agent meaning cell-damaging)
- No healing or detoxing practices in her lifestyle

I will guide you in identifying these factors and things that you can do to change them. We will go through the Keeping Well journey together by learning about the body and its ability to heal. I will help you ward off cancer to the best of your ability with diet and lifestyle changes. Most importantly we will do this while keeping a positive outlook on life. After all, you, not the cancer, are in the driver's seat now.

"An ounce of prevention is worth a pound of cure."
— Benjamin Franklin

It's one thing to study natural therapies, but meeting people firsthand who have healed themselves from terminal cancer is a life-changing experience. I attended The Truth About Cancer conference in 2017, which had over forty of the most renowned cancer and natural health experts in attendance. The audience was a mix of cancer patients, survivors, health practitioners, and curious health-conscious people looking to learn more. Within fifteen minutes of getting there, I had met many survivors, some of whom had been diagnosed with "terminal" cancer. The most incredible part was that they all healed in different ways. They incorporated holistic practices to their medical treatment such as; naturopathy, herbs, juicing, vegan and keto diets, to name a few. The body truly wants to heal itself you just have to give it the right tools, and there are many tools to do so. In this book, we will dive into preventative healing practices and lifestyle changes you can make to reduce your risk of cancer and heal the body from the toxic load of this modern world.

My wish for you is to take everything that resonates with you and leave what doesn't. You know your body best, and your intuition knows your body even better. Use your first initial instinct before the logical mind kicks in to know what practices are calling to you. Everyone is different and some of the practices in this book might not appeal to you. Use this guide to discover what your body is asking for.

Chapter 3:

I AM KEEPING MY BODY WELL BY LISTENING TO WHAT IT HAS TO SAY

"Believe you can and you're halfway there."
– Theodore Roosevelt

The problem with the Western medicine philosophy on treating cancer is that it does not address the root cause. As an analogy, you can cut (surgery), burn (radiation), or poison (chemotherapy) a weed, but if the root is deep enough, it will come back sooner or later. Western medicine often treats the symptoms rather than the cause. This could explain why many people, like my mom, get cancer again years after they went into remission. My hope is that this book helps you create a sustainable anti-cancer, healthy lifestyle that addressed the root cause of cancer. I will guide you in determining the cancer-causing factors in your life, give you the information on how to change them, and then set you up with an eight-week plan to keeping well.

Identifying the causative factors of why you got sick in the first place is your key to healing. If you had a bacterial infection, the doctor would do a lab test to see what strain of bacteria was causing the problem and then give you an antibiotic that works to kill that specific strain. Identify the causative factors to your health problem and work accordingly to correct them. To know the cause is to know the cure. I love this saying, but I do hate the word cure. To me, it implies that one day there will be a magical pill or shot that will prevent people from getting cancer. That would be great, but the "war on cancer" has been going on since President Nixon signed the National Cancer Act of 1971, about forty years ago. Death rates have declined, but cancer still affects over one million people in the United States every year. To turn the odds in your favor requires a lifestyle change that goes against the one that made you sick in the first place.

Some causes of cancer include inherited genetics, chronic inflammation, stress, nutritional factors, immune disorders, chronic infections, and iatrogenic (illness caused by medical treatment, like chemo-induced cancer).

Genetics give us a predisposition to certain types of illnesses, but genes can be turned on and off by environmental triggers. You may have a genetic predisposition to breast cancer yet have a healthy lifestyle that never "turns on" that gene. You are not a slave to your genetics; you have a solid upper hand in how they play out.

By having a healthy lifestyle that takes into account nutrition and emotional wellness, you also have the upper hand when it comes to the remaining causative factors. An anti-cancer diet is one with lots of fruits and vegetables and very limited inflammatory substances like processed food and alcohol. This reduces inflammation in the body, balances nutrition, heals the body from past abuse (like chemotherapy), and can even help with chronic infections. Chronic infections include an overgrowth of microorganisms like bacteria, viruses, yeast (candida), fungi, mold, and parasites. Fruits, vegetables, and herbs contain substances that help to naturally combat these. When you look at the big picture it just makes sense, right? Your health comes down to your inherited genetic weaknesses, environmental factors, emotional status, what you eat, and what you eliminate.

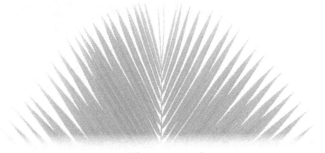

Chapter 4:

I UNDERSTAND HOW MY BODY WORKS, SO I KNOW HOW TO HEAL IT

B efore I guide you into keeping well, there are a few body systems you need to understand first. I will guide you through the functions of the skin, lymphatic, and digestive systems, including specifically that of the kidneys and liver, using a holistic approach. You will learn how they work to detox your body and how to assist them in this job.

You can't fix it if you didn't read the manual. Most humans have no idea how to work their machines. Just the word anatomy might take you over the edge, but before I lose you, I promise this is going to be the easiest class you've ever taken. Basic human anatomy is quite simple, learning the names of 650 muscles and 206 bones, not so much. No tests today, but I promise you will gain so much value from this detox anatomy 101 class.

Basic human anatomy as it relates to detoxification and healing the body.

Skin

Let's work our way in and start with the skin. Did you know that the skin is the largest organ of your body? Consider the skin a low-permeability sponge rather than a shield of armor from the outside world. Dermal absorption can transport chemicals from the surface into the body. The body is capable of absorbing products depending on the molecular size – for example, the aluminum in commercial deodorant, which has been found in breast tissue. So, when it comes to the skin, you can have your cake and eat it too – if you're using a vanilla cupcake–scented body lotion that is.

What an abused organ the skin has become. It has been peacefully doing its job of protection, regulation, and sensation since the beginning of time. Then along came the daily dose of chemical-scented body washes, lotions, makeup, and perfumes. Regular exposure to everyday things like body wash might seem trivial, but the average woman unknowingly applies 126 chemical ingredients from personal care products per day according to the EWG. In just one year, that cumulative ingredient exposure totals 45,990. A study published in the American Journal of Public Health showed that an average of 64% of what you put on your skin is absorbed into the bloodstream. Products applied to the underarms can have an absorption rate of 100%. Let's make sure you're using the good stuff instead.[3] These are several natural product lines that work great and also smell amazing; Andalou, Passport to Organics, Skincado, Symmetrie Oils, and Tikkun Illume. The last three lines are made by dear friends who put their heart into the products they make, and it truly shows!

I have been in the skincare industry all of my adult life. Since I became an esthetician at nineteen, I have seen firsthand how the market has taken off in the direction of natural beauty products. It is truly incredible and a much-needed change. When I was in school ten years ago for skin care, there was little to no education on the benefit of using organic and natural products. Even the products we used in school contained parabens. Parabens are used as a preservative in personal care products. They have been linked to breast cancer due to their estrogen-mimicking ability, which causes hormone disruption. While the European Union has banned five different parabens (isopropylparaben, isobutylparaben, phenylparaben, benzylparaben, and pentylparaben), the FDA in the United States has not. Unfortunately, the same goes for more than one thousand ingredients that the European Union has banned in cosmetics and the United States has not.

Shop safer by avoiding the ingredients below.

Fragrance

What is fragrance? Also listed as perfume and parfum, it's one word that is in the ingredient list of almost all commercial beauty products. What hides behind this one word can be up to one hundred different unnamed chemical ingredients. This loophole was created to protect fragrance trade secrets. The chemical components of fragrance are hidden so that trademarked fragrances cannot be copied. Fragrance is one of the most common reasons people have allergic reactions to cosmetic products.

Phthalates

Commonly found in skin care, hair care, soaps, and other body products, phthalates have been banned in the European Union, but their use is still common in the United States. According to the CDC, measurable levels of phthalate metabolytes have been found in the general population but are highest in women. They are banned in the EU for their harmful effect on the reproductive system.[4]

Aluminum

Aluminum salts are used in commercial deodorants to prevent sweat and kill bacteria. It can penetrate the skin and has been found in breast tissue. Daily exposure burdens the body with this nonessential metal. Aluminum's ability to prevent sweat is also of concern since sweat is our body's way of getting rid of toxins. Anything that hinders the body's ability to detox daily should be of concern. This is your body's natural defense to keeping itself clean. By not sweating you are keeping the toxic burden inside of you for the lymphatic system and other organs to deal with. More on this further along.

There are many great natural deodorant brands that actually work, and trust me, it has been quite the trial and error for me to tell you this. My two favorite brands are Each and Every and Lavanila. The cleaner the body is, the less it will smell. You will notice the more you sweat and cleaner foods you eat, the less you smell. Aim to break a sweat once a day. You can do this through working out, using a sauna, or taking a hot Epsom salt bath. Most people have been using conventional deodorant all of their lives. To detox the armpit from years of deodorant abuse, apply a paste made from bentonite clay and water for twenty minutes a week. Bentonite clay helps to draw impurities from the skin. If you choose to keep wearing conventional deodorant with aluminum, then at least remove it before you go to bed.

Sodium Lauryl Sulfate

Commonly found in shampoo, body wash, and toothpaste, SLS is an irritating surfactant that makes products foam up. It is known to be a skin irritant because of its ability to strip the skin of its vital oils and cause dry skin. I added this to the list because even though it is not a harmful chemical, it disrupts the skin on a regular basis.

BHA + BHT

Butylated hydroxyanisole (BHA) and butylated hydroxytoluene (BHT) are used as preservatives in food and cosmetics. They are shown to be possible human carcinogens (cancer-promoting) and endocrine disrupters. You can find them in many kinds of cereal, chips, and body care products.

The skin is also a good reflection of your internal state of health – as above, so below, as the saying goes. When the skin shows problems like rashes, eczema, psoriasis, dry skin, and acne, it is often a sign of deeper issues within the body. The skin is an eliminatory organ and will push out toxins through the skin if the liver, kidneys, lymphatic system, and digestive tract are taxed. From now on think of the body as one big system of cause and effect.

For example, when the kidneys can't filter waste from the blood effectively, the skin will supplement and sweat out its uric acid waste onto the skin. High levels of this uric acid are commonly found in patients with the skin condition psoriasis.[5] Kidney disease is more likely in people with severe psoriasis. Finally, patients with gout (uric acid in the joints) experience a higher prevalence of psoriasis. Uric acid is a substance formed when the body breaks down purines. Some foods responsible for high purine include meat, seafood, sugar, fast food, and alcohol. Your body is simply one big system of cause and effect. Fix the cause factors before there's an effect.

Skin, Sun, and Cancer

When it comes to sun exposure it is important to find a happy medium. Too much exposure damages the skin, yet too little can cause a vitamin D deficiency. Vitamin D is made when the skin is exposed to sunlight. When it comes to breast cancer, research suggests that women with low levels of vitamin D have a higher risk. "Vitamin D may play a role in controlling normal breast cell growth and may be able to stop breast cancer cells from growing."[6] Aside from breast cancer, low levels have correlated with several cancers, including colorectal, kidney, lung, and pancreatic.[7]

When you think of your average day, how often are you exposed to sunlight? For most, it's just a quick peek here and there, probably getting out of the car going to and from places. Now, of course I want you to get responsible exposure by avoiding peak hours (roughly 11:00 a.m. to 2:00 p.m.) and using a natural sunblock. My recommendation is to sit outside with your morning smoothie for five minutes a day, taking in the morning low-index sunlight while getting your daily dose of hydration and nutrients.

When it comes to sunscreen, I recommend a non-chemical formula that uses mineral blockers instead. From a common-sense point of view, does covering your dear skin in a chemical sunblock along with the perfume smell (more chemicals) and then baking in the sun sound like a good idea? There's a better way. Chemical-free sunscreens use minerals as their active ingredient instead. Look for zinc oxide or titanium dioxide as the active ingredient on the label.

What's so harmful about most commercial sunblock? Well, the FDA has found that four of the most common active chemical ingredients in commercial sunblock can be absorbed through the skin and into the body. While the effects of these chemicals are unknown, a simple switch will help you to be safe and not sorry.[8]

Active Ingredients to Avoid:
- Oxybenzone
- Octocrylene
- Avobenzone

Anti-Cancer Skincare Tips:

- Avoid anything with fragrance in the ingredient list. Thanks to trade law secrets, the chemical composure of fragrance doesn't need to be listed. Which means this one word, fragrance, can contain hundreds of chemicals that do not have to be labeled.
- Download the Think Dirty App to get an instant safety rating of any cosmetic product you are about to buy just by scanning its barcode.
- Exfoliate with a full-body scrub once a week. Skin cells rejuvenate slower with age.
- Use a shower filter to eliminate tap water contaminants. A shower filter also reduces the amount of inhaled pollutants from tap water taken in from the shower vapor. You can see what contaminants are in your tap water using your zip code and the EWG Tap Water Database: https://www.ewg.org/tapwater/
- Steam saunas are great for skin detoxification. You can get a small personal size steam sauna on Amazon for around $100.
- Add magnesium salt baths to your routine regularly. Magnesium baths are good for stress relief, skin problems, and mineral absorption. They also help you sleep

better. A hot magnesium bath makes the body sweat, which is a great toxin release for the skin.

- Bentonite clay baths help to draw toxins and potentially radiation from the body. I do a hot bath with one to two cups of bentonite clay for twenty minutes once a week. Bentonite clay has been shown to act as a detoxifying agent because of its absorption capacity.

In the back of this book is a link to my website for all my favorite personal care products.

Lymphatic System

Learning how the lymphatic system works is a pillar to understanding how to improve your health because it plays a significant role in waste elimination and protection. Lymph is the main fluid in your body next to blood. In my work, I also find that this is the least understood system of the body. Here's how it works.

The fish tank analogy. What happens to a fish tank if the filter stops working? It gets cloudy and dirty. The same thing happens to your body when you're stationary. You know how you are about 60% water? Well that water gets dirty from cellular waste. Every day you and your cells are eating and eliminating. The fluid system in your body does not have a pump like your blood does (the heart). It requires your bodies movement via muscular contractions to move the fluid in your body to the lymph nodes which acts as a sewer system, cleaning the debris and bacteria in the lymph (body fluid) and returning it cleaned to the body just like that fish tank filter.

Just like our circulatory system of arteries and veins, there are lymphatic veins and ducts. Instead of having a central meeting point like the heart as the circulatory system does, they empty to the nearest lymph node. There are lymph nodes all throughout the body, especially the neck, armpit, and groin area.

The lymphatic capillaries and vessels run all around the body adjunct to the blood vessels and arteries. Their job is to gather and clean the fluid in your body. The capillaries are permeable to collect this body fluid that contains debris from inside the body like cell waste, dead cells, proteins, cancer cells, bacteria, and pathogens. If there has been any damage or harm to the body like cancer, they become more permeable to gather the excess debris to keep the body fluid clean before returning to the blood.

From the lymph capillaries and vessels, this fluid passes through the lymph nodes where it is cleaned and filtered by our immune system. Your immune system provides white blood cells to kill everything that doesn't belong, such as foreign particles, bacteria, viruses, and cancer cells. They engulf the debris and work to dissolve or break them down into small harmless particles. Finally, the cleaned body fluid is ready to enter into your blood.

Have you have ever felt a swollen nodule around your throat when you get sick? That is simply the lymph node doing its job as part of the immune system to engulf the bacteria or virus that is making you sick.

The lymphatic system needs our help to do its job. Unlike the blood, this fluid system does not have a pump like the heart. It relies solely on our movement via exercise and deep breathing. The lymph vessels get squeezed by our muscular contractions and the pressure of our breaths.

Exercise and deep breathing are key components to keeping the lymphatic system clean and moving. Find a type of movement you love. My favorite is barre classes. It's a workout I look forward to and love! Try new things until you find a type of movement that you also love! Get those muscles contracting and pushing that body fluid to the filters to get cleaned.

What damages the lymphatic system? Chronic high-fat diets impair lymphatic function. When you eat fat, it's absorbed from the digestive system into the lymph. Can you imagine how much effort it takes the body to pump bacon grease through tiny vessels? The healthier and cleaner we eat, the easier the job our lymphatic system has.[9]

Liver

The liver, no lie, has more than a thousand functions. As you can imagine, it is pretty essential to keep this organ working well. Its primary duties include metabolizing protein, carbs, and fat. It also stores and converts amino acids (building blocks of protein), glucose, various vitamins, and minerals. All the food and drinks you have must be broken down into its simplest form for your body to absorb and use. The further from nature you eat, the harder your body works to break down and utilize its components.

Under your liver is the gallbladder, which stores the bile produced by the liver. Bile is used during digestion as an alkalizer, anti-inflammatory agent, and fat emulsifier. It works to break down large fat molecules, regulates inflammation, and reduces acids during early-stage digestion.

Given this information, you can conclude to reduce taxation on the gallbladder you should:

- Stay away from unhealthy fats (fried foods)
- Eat an anti-inflammatory and alkaline-dominant diet (whole foods)

Occasionally I see this meme online that drives me crazy. It's a picture of the liver that says, "You don't need to do a detox; you have a liver" – as if the liver is a mystical creature capable of putting up with extraordinary tasks. Give it a break, literally. A healthy liver is capable of detoxifying hormones (like birth control), drugs, toxins, and alcohol, but how much abuse is too much abuse? A damaged liver may not be able to process as many toxins.

Kidneys

The kidneys are connected to the bladder. They filter the blood and eliminate excess water, nutrients, and waste from the body through urine. First the liver breaks down substances and makes waste water-soluble so the kidneys can excrete it. Staying properly hydrated is an import part of eliminating toxins from the body. I like to follow the rule of having half your body weight in ounces of water a day. So if you weigh 160 pounds, then you should drink eighty ounces of water a day. Hydration can also come from having lots of water-rich, fresh fruits and vegetables in your diet.

Urine contains byproducts of your metabolism, some of which include urea acid, ammonia, creatine, medications, toxins, and pesticides. This toxic waste is stored in the bladder on a daily basis. If you have very acidic and toxic waste in your urine from unhealthy eating and drinking, what do you think this is doing to the integrity of your bladder?

Digestion System

The body is built from what you eat during your lifetime. All of your cells are continually taking in nutrients and excreting out waste. What are you feeding them, and can they eliminate the waste properly? You can be either building and repairing the body with abundant nutrients or burdening it with junk.

The digestive system includes the mouth, stomach, and small and large intestine. I purposely put this system last. I think first understanding the lymphatic system, kidney, and liver helps you better connect how digestion affects the entire body. There are three key factors when it comes to digestion: how well do you digest food, absorb its nutrients, and eliminate its waste byproducts.

Digestion starts in the mouth. I can't stress how important it is to chew your food enough. If you have any problems with digestion, analyze how well you chew your food. The body doesn't magically break down un-chewed pieces of food without a large amount of effort and enzymes. Have you ever felt tired after a large meal? That is because digestion uses most of your body's energy. Save some energy and chew your food. The saliva excretes the enzyme amylase, which breaks down starches and carbohydrates. If you aren't chewing starchy foods well enough, you are missing out on a key component to their digestion.

Absorption takes place largely in the small intestine, which is the first, and longest, part of the bowel. The walls of the small intestine are covered with tiny little finger-like projections called villi. These projections give more surface area for nutrients to be absorbed by the blood and lymph. The nutrients absorbed into the blood from the small intestine goes right to the liver for detoxification and filtering.

After the small intestine, food enters the large intestine, also called the colon. The colon is about five feet long, and it is where any remaining water and nutrients are absorbed, making the waste solid. The colon needs the proper amount of fiber to work effectively. Fiber is the indigestible parts of plants and grains that provide bulk to our stool; it helps remaining waste to be pushed along the digestive tract like a mop. Low-fiber diets are associated with colon cancer. Low fiber foods include meat, dairy, white bread and pastas, eggs, and most junk foods. Sounds like the typical standard American diet (SAD). If you aren't getting enough cleaning from fiber acting like a mop in the colon and moving things along, then the food matter is sitting in the colon rotting away. Colon hydrotherapy, also known as colonics, helps to remove this old waste and is a good tool to have on hand when transitioning to healthier lifestyle.

Probiotics

Your gut has a complex microbiome and when it is in balance things run smoothly. The colon has a population of good bacteria that help to break down undigested food, absorb nutrients, produce vitamin K, keep you regular, and support the immune system. These good bacteria are called probiotics.

Things that disrupt this delicate balance and kill probiotics include; alcohol, poor diet, chemotherapy, and antibiotics. With an unbalanced gut you may experience constipation, digestive problems, skin conditions, and moodiness to name a few. It is important to work on fixing your gut especially after chemotherapy.

A healthy gut starts with a healthy diet filled with fruit, vegetables, and grains which have dietary fiber that is essential to feeding this good bacteria. A plant heavy diet and taking a probiotic supplement will help to bring the good bacteria into proper balance again. As it relates to cancer, taking a probiotic supplement has been found to help with chemotherapy-induced diarrhea. Having this healthy, good bacteria is essential for optimal digestion and health.

Proper Food Combining for Optimal Health

Certain foods digest and leave the stomach differently. Fruits and vegetables digest and leave the stomach quickest, followed by carbohydrates, and lastly denser protein and fat meals. For optimal digestion, I recommend eating light to heavy. This means eating easier to digest foods in the morning like fruits, followed by a light lunch, and a heavier meal for dinner. My friend Shannon, a colon hydrotherapist of nine years, always says the first thing you eat in the morning sets the tone for the day. I find this to be true over and over again. If you start the morning with a super hydrating, easy to digest smoothie, then you are more likely to crave lighter and healthier foods throughout the day. If you start the morning with a bagel or something dense, you continue to crave heavier and heavier foods throughout the day. Analyze what you start your day with and what you crave throughout the day afterward. You will be so surprised at how this holds true.

Fruits should be eaten alone or left alone. Fruits are super simple for the body to digest. They should be eaten in the morning or when you have an empty stomach. Imagine if you just had a burger with lots of protein, fat, and carbs and then have a fruit salad for dessert. Once you eat that fruit, it is ready to go for digestion, but there's a big, juicy burger in the way. So the fruit sits in the digestive system for longer than it needs. This poses a problem because it is fermenting and sitting in the digestive system for longer than it should.

Protein and starches should not be eaten together. I know this can be a hard one to work with given it is the basic dinner plate. However, protein and starches need two different enzymes for digestion in the stomach. So when eating these, digestive mediums neutralize each other, and it takes much longer for the pair to digest than it would if they were eaten separately. Have you ever been sleepy after having a large plate of food? That is due to the amount of energy the body is using for digestion. Proper food combing can help save some of this much-needed energy for more important tasks like healing and repairing.

The pancreas is what secrets digestive enzymes into the small intestine to break down food, as well as secreting insulin and glucagon to control the blood sugar in the blood.

I like to give clients the slow-cooker example. Imagine a slow cooker set to 98.6 degrees. As you eat throughout the day, you add the food to the slow cooker. This is a simple visualization you can do to analyze your digestion and see what may be causing problems. Let's say you just had two slices of cheese pizza for dinner, but you were thirsty, so you had a glass of orange juice afterward. The orange juice meets the cheese pizza in the slow cooker, aka your stomach, at about 98.6 degrees. Normally the orange juice would be in and out, but there's a cheese pizza that the stomach is trying to digest. The orange juice is mixing around with the yeast from the pizza crust and fermenting away at nearly 100 degrees for at least an hour. Yikes. Bring on the indigestion, bloating, and acid reflux from this acidic sludge. Water may have been a better choice.

Optimal Digestion Cheat Sheet

- Fruits, juices, and smoothies should be eaten alone and on an empty stomach

- Starches and proteins should be eaten separately
- Combining fats and starches are okay
- Combining vegetables and starches are okay
- Combining vegetables and proteins are okay
- Combining fruit and vegetables are generally okay
- Melons should always be eaten alone
- Heavier, harder to digest foods should be eaten at the end of the day
- Black pepper helps with digestion
- Taking a probiotic in the morning helps to balance gut bacteria for good digestion
- Take a digestive enzyme if you had a cheat meal or improper food combination

Pesticides versus Organic

A huge reason to eat organic food is to maintain the integrity of your intestinal wall. When the wall is impaired, causing malabsorption, you don't get the nutrients from food. A study on fish exposed to the popular pesticide glyphosate showed the development of digestive problems that are reminiscent of celiac disease.[10] Celiac disease is a disorder that affects the lining of the small intestine, causing inflammation and preventing proper absorption, which leads to vitamin and mineral deficiencies. It also causes abdominal pain, bloating, fatigue, diarrhea, headaches, anemia, and many more symptoms. The popular pesticide glyphosate has also recently been found to significantly increase the risk of non-Hodgkin lymphoma, a cancer of the immune system. Reducing pesticides in the diet is a sure way to maintain the integrity of your body.

A few years ago, I accidentally learned how harmful pesticides can be. I was living in an apartment where the landscaping was taken care of by the development during the day when I was at work. At the time I had two cats who loved to be outside on the patio and grass. Can you see where this is going? I would let my cat, Ace, out to explore whenever I was outside. He loved to roll around in the grass by my patio. A few months after living there he started getting open sores, some bigger than a quarter, on different areas of his body. After a $500 vet bill, many tests, blood work, and steroids they told me they didn't know what was wrong. They gave me a topical solution to apply to help heal the sores and sent me on my way with a monthly follow-up. The following week, I was lying outside reading a book on my patio when all of a sudden, I heard a spraying noise coming toward me. When I looked up, there was a landscaper in a full protective body suit spraying pesticides around everyone's patios. Immediately I knew why my cat was developing raw open sores all over his body. He enjoyed rolling around right where they sprayed on a regular basis. Guess what? After realizing he was rolling around in pesticides, I banned him from going outside. After a month, he stopped getting the sores and has not had them since.

If organic food is unavailable to you for any reason, there is a rule of thumb you can follow for reducing pesticide exposure. Some produce is more concentrated in pesticides than others, depending on the skin of the fruit and farming. Fruit and veggies with outer skin that you peel away, like watermelon and pineapple, don't expose you to as much pesticide residue because you are peeling away the potentially sprayed skin. Fruits and veggies that don't have a skin you dispose of, like peaches, lettuce, and berries, should be bought organic whenever possible. You are eating where the pesticides were sprayed. Even if they have been washed very well, you have to think, do pesticide chemicals sit on top of the lettuce and get washed away? Or can a pesticide chemical potentially soak into the lettuce? Again, it is better to be safe than sorry when it comes to your health. Below is a list of fruits and vegetables that should be bought organic and a list that can be bought nonorganic depending on pesticide residue.

Buy organic:
- Berries
- Lettuce
- Peaches
- Plums

- Apples
- Pears
- Grapes
- Celery
- Potatoes
- Peppers
- Tomatoes

OK to buy nonorganic:
- Melons
- Pineapple
- Broccoli
- Cauliflower
- Avocados
- Corn
- Papaya
- Kiwi
- Onions
- Squash

"Disease is not the presence of something evil,
but rather the lack of the presence
of something essential."
– Dr. Bernard Jensen

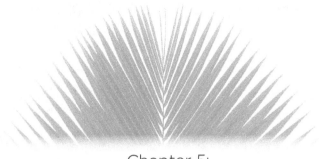

Chapter 5:

I KNOW MY BODY HAS THE ABILITY TO HEAL ITSELF AND I ASSIST IT IN EVERY WAY

*"The food you eat can be either the safest
and most powerful form of medicine
or the slowest form of poison."*
- Ann Wigmore

B y first learning how the body works, you can for the rest of your life make decisions that support its functions. If you can't tell by now, I like to be as easygoing as possible when it comes to maintaining a healthy lifestyle. I want you to have all the tools to live a healthy life while still enjoying life to the fullest because that is what it's all about.

You probably expected the nutrition chapter of this book to be the longest. You're in for a treat because it is going to be one of the shortest chapters. It is that simple of a topic when you understand the foundational pillars. People get so caught up in what to eat and what not to eat. When you look at the big picture, it is so simple. I follow a plant-based diet free of animal products and mostly whole, unprocessed foods. That works best for me, and I will briefly touch on the health effects of meat and dairy. However; I do believe in doing what works for you. Everyone is different. The rules below can be adapted to meat-eaters and vegans alike.

The Eighty/Twenty Rule

There is an easy rule to remember what to eat to maintain an anti-cancer lifestyle. It is the eighty/twenty rule. It is easy to remember and will ensure optimal vitality through proper nutrition. When thinking of your diet as a pie chart, envision these ratios when eating throughout the day.

80% — Clean food that is unprocessed and health-promoting.
20% — Processed and acidic foods such as; white flours, sugar, dairy, meat, caffeine, and alcohol.

The daily goal is to bring this as close as you can to 100 percent clean foods.

Addressing Animal Products

I know many people reading this are not ready to give up eating meat completely, and I support that. As mentioned earlier, I recommend keeping it in the minimal to 20 percent category if you do. This is because the World Health Organization has classified processed meat as a Group 1 carcinogen to humans. This means that there is sufficient evidence that meat is cancer-causing to humans based on its connection to colon cancer. To put this into perspective, smoking and asbestos are also in this Group 1 classification. Crazy right?[11]

This classification is specifically for processed meat like hotdogs, lunch meats, bacon, salami, and sausages. There is also strong correlation for cancer risk and red meat, especially for colon, pancreatic, and prostate cancer.

If continuing to eat meat, I would urge to choose hormone- and antibiotic-free options. Choose grass-fed if you are still eating red meat and wild-caught if you are still eating fish. Fish is a large source of pollutants, radiation, and heavy metals. Just eat accordingly.

When it comes to dairy, I again say to avoid it or keep it in the minimal to twenty percent category. To put it simply, you just don't need it. Dairy is breast milk from cows that are meant to turn a baby cow into a thousand-pound adult within a short amount of time. Dairy contains IGF-1, a hormone that helps cells grow. Cancer is an abnormal growth of cells that proliferate in an uncontrolled way. See how this could be a problem? Studies show that having higher IGF-1 levels can increase the development of certain cancers like prostate, breast, and colorectal.[12]

So, What Do I Eat?

"Fruits for electricity,
Vegetables for grounding,
Herbs for healing,
Nuts + seeds for building."
– Dr. Sebi

Simply put, follow the rules in this chapter and eat a diet of mostly organic fruits, vegetables, whole grains, plant-based protein, and healthy fats.

When eating sugar, think: Do I want to feed the bacteria and yeast in my body?

When drinking soda, think: Do I want to tax my kidneys by putting this acidic fluid in my body?

When eating junk food, think: Do I want to tax my digestive and lymphatic system with this processed oil?

One of my favorite memories now is when my mom found out about two anti-cancer foods. She heard some anti-cancer health tips probably from a TV show like Dr. Oz. One was that white tea is the highest in antioxidants and is good for cancer patients. Needless to say, she had white tea almost every day after that. Another was when she found out that bok choy is an anti-cancer food as well. There was bok choy in the fridge every day after that. What makes me cringe ten years later as a detox specialist is that she added bok choy and carrots to a ramen noodle packet as an easy soup recipe. I'm talking about the Maruchan instant ramen soup in the orange package that costs about ninety-nine cents and has preservatives, nonorganic wheat flour, MSG, sugar, and more sodium than you should have in a week. She had good intentions, but education just wasn't there. If only I could have handed her this chapter!

"Your health is what you make of it. Everything you do and think either adds to the vitality, energy, and spirit you possess or takes away from it."

— Ann Wigmore

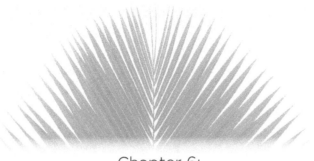

Chapter 6:

I CREATE A HEALTHY ENVIRONMENT ALL AROUND ME

"You cannot heal in the same environment where you got sick."
- Unknown

Your external environment reflects your internal one. If your environment is full of toxins, so are you. Do these invisible toxins we can't see impact our risk for cancer? The Halifax Project is one of the best studies to see this because it tested the carcinogenic effect of low-dose chemicals we encounter in the environment. Not only that, but it also took into account the effects of the combination of these chemicals on our health. Governmental agencies test for the safety of chemicals, but rarely do they test the safety of multiple chemicals combined. The Halifax Project found that of the eighty-five common chemicals not known to be carcinogenic on their own, fifty of them, when in combination with others and at low doses encountered in the environment, can disrupt cancer-related pathways.[13]

There are just so many unknowns when it comes to chemicals. So why not just do what we can to minimize our exposure to them, especially in our home environment? The following is a guide to reducing the chemical cocktails in our daily external environment.

Creating a Healthy Environment:

Air

The biggest space in our house is the air. We can't see it, so it's often overlooked when it comes to our health and healing environment. We also spend most of our time indoors, and the air quality at home can be five times more polluted than outdoors. The Environmental Protection Agency states indoor air pollution is America's number-one environmental health problem.

Anything that irritates our body creates inflammation, so reducing air pollutants and allergens is one step to reducing chronic inflammation. Luckily, changing a few things can make a huge difference in our indoor air quality.

Indoor pollutants you may be exposed to include; dust, mold, mildew, pet allergens, dust mites, smoke, bacteria, viruses, carpet and furniture off-gases, cleaning supplies, and fragrance. I recommend getting an indoor air filter. I have the Air Doctor air filter, and I love it. Let me tell you, if you think the air filter in your HVAC is enough, you have not seen the filter in my Air Doctor. This is especially good if you have pets, to prevent pet allergens.

A few natural alternatives to eliminate some common pollutants include switching your candles out with a plant-based alternative that is scented with essential oils instead of fragrance. Most candles are petroleum-based. So you are essentially burning fossil fuel every time you light a candle. Think car exhaust. Multiple studies have found "fragrance" to be a known human immune toxicant and allergen. Have you ever walked down the laundry aisle and started coughing or having burning eyes? Or perhaps walked past the perfume section of the department store and had a similar reaction? That would be a high dose of fragrance in action. I like to make a DIY room and linen spray by mixing a few drops of essential oil into a spray bottle of rose water. The Heritage Store brand is my favorite affordable rose water spray. I like to add a few drops of cinnamon essential oil for its antibacterial properties. Some other good ones to try are lemon and lavender essential oil.

A big indoor pollutant is toxic cleaning products. Try replacing chemical cleaning supplies with natural alternatives. I know this will be a hard one for some people, but I'm telling you my life has not been the same since I discovered Norwex. I recommend watching some YouTube videos on how to use their products as they do require some explaining. They are by far the cleanest and most effective products I have ever found. I love their microfiber cloths which are infused with silver for its antimicrobial properties. You are essentially cleaning with water when you use them. Trust me: look them up.

Water

Remember the Erin Brockovich movie with Julia Roberts where she found a cancer-causing chemical in tap water? That was twenty-six years ago back in 1993 and she won a case against Pacific Gas & Electric in California. Well that cancer-causing chemical, chromium-6, is still found in the tap water of more than 200 million Americans in all fifty states. Crazy right? The California scientists set a so-called public health goal of 0.02 parts per billion in tap water, the level that would pose negligible risk over a lifetime of consumption. That's our singular lifetime.

Remember the Pottenger cat experiment from Chapter 1? We are down one generation since then. Exposure to chromium-6 can lead to lung cancer, liver damage, reproductive problems, and developmental harm.[14]

If you get anything from this book, let it be to just never drink tap water, please. Here are some means of protecting ourselves from the mysterious "safe levels" of various chemicals that infiltrate tap water.

Get a shower filter. Don't even wait to save up for an expensive top-of-the-line one. Buy a fifteen-dollar one from your local Home Depot and start using it in the meantime. Your skin and hair will thank you. Tap water is treated with chlorine to kill dangerous bacteria, so you probably drink chlorine every single day. Chlorine kills bacteria, but we have plenty of good bacteria in our bodies that need to be there to keep balance, especially for good digestion. Our skin is a sponge, so when showering, we drink in that water and its contaminants. We also breathe it in the chlorine vapor, especially if you enjoy long, hot, steamy showers.

Get a water filter for drinking water. I use an inexpensive forty-dollar Zero Water filter that I bought from Target and it has been great. It holds thirty cups of water in a ready-to-dispense container, so you don't have to refill it constantly. It comes with a PPM tester, which tests the parts per million of dissolved solids in the water. My tap water is about 155 PPM, and after you use the filter, it is 0 PPM. It removes the chlorine, sediment, metals, lead, chromium, and hydrogen sulfide, to name a few. There are plenty of water filters even better than the Zero Water brand on the market. I'm just telling you the one I currently use and love. I don't care which one you buy, as long as you buy one so that you are not having trace amounts of the contaminants listed above. This has greatly reduced my plastic water bottle usage (I have a few glass bottles and a steel HydraPeak that I love), which is another step towards an anti-cancer lifestyle. Chemicals from plastic leach into our food, especially if the plastic is heated in any way. So never drink out of a water bottle that was left in a hot car. We've banned BPA from many plastic goods already for mimicking estrogen in our body, but do we know much about its replacements? A new study finds "Bisphenol S (BPS), a substitute for the chemical bisphenol A (BPA) in the plastic industry, shows the potential for increasing the aggressiveness of breast cancer through its behavior as an endocrine-disrupting chemical."[15]

Radiation

Let's take a look at another invisible contaminant, Wi-Fi. A study found exposure to radio frequency radiation emitted from Wi-Fi caused impaired insulin secretion and increased oxidative stress in rat pancreatic islets.[16] Another study done on rats showed evidence of oxidative stress after continuous exposure to Wi-Fi radiation where a significant decrease was detected in total antioxidant capacity of plasma and the activities of several antioxidant enzymes.[17] Wi-Fi and cell phone radiation, which are essentially the same thing, just haven't been around long enough to know its true impact on our health. This is something we are around 24/7, especially if you live in densely populated areas. Do you ever turn your Wi-Fi router off? Probably not, right? I have had a Wi-Fi router on in my house since the beginning of non-dial-up internet. Only this year, twenty years later, have I started to unplug my Wi-Fi router when it's not in use. That is a twenty-year experiment that our generation is the guinea pigs for.

I also recommend not sleeping close to your cell phone and reducing your use of Bluetooth technology when you can. Putting your phone on airplane mode when you're sleeping is the most radiation reducing thing you can do aside from turning it off. Just make sure you turn the airplane mode off when you wake up or you will not receive calls or texts.

Chapter 7

I WELCOME ALL EMOTIONS TO BE HEALED

*"You cannot have a positive life
and a negative mind."*
- Joyce Meyer

So far, you've learned about healing the physical body through food and detoxification, but there is one thing missing when it comes to true healing: the emotional and mental body. You are much more than just a physical body. True healing comes when body, mind, and emotions are all in harmony. There are many ways in which your emotions affect your physical health so let's get those thoughts in a positive direction to ensure optimal health.

The physical body is simply the shell that houses all that we are: our emotions, mind, and soul. It runs on autopilot and is a self-regulating machine if we provide it with the right fuel. Just like a car, it requires proper fuel (diet), occasional maintenance (detox), and regular use (exercise) to keep it running at its best. You are the driver of your body and your emotions can steer the wheel.

Did you know when you cry, you are releasing hormones in your tears, therefore excreting them whole rather than using your liver to metabolize them? It is a physical discharge of emotion. Cry it out if you need to. Alternatively, laughter can promote healing in the body by decreasing stress hormones. It also increases blood flow, releases endorphins, and boosts the immune system.

The mind creates emotions, and the cells of your body physically respond to emotions. The mind composes your thoughts of the past, present, and future. The body can heal and restore itself only when it is calm and relaxed in a parasympathetic state. Stressing about future events that haven't happened yet or reliving stressful events from the past keep the body in a sympathetic, fight or flight state. For example, if you are in a state of stress, your body goes into fight or flight mode. The adrenal glands produce adrenaline to give you added strength to combat the task at hand. Humans today live in a chronic state of stress because of the busy-ness of modern-day life. This chronic stressed state causes anxiety and prevents the body from healing and restoring. You cannot be stressed and healing at the same time. Some powerful healing methods to balance the physical and emotional body include; crying, laughing, meditating, practicing gratitude, trying energy healing, practicing yoga, getting some time in nature, and talking to a friend. Take a moment to write down ten things you are grateful for.

How emotions affect organs:
- Anger affects the liver
- Grief affects the lungs
- Worry/ Stress affects the stomach
- Stress affects the nervous system
- Fear affects the kidneys
- Heartache/ Betrayal affects the heart
- Anxiety/ Weight of the world affects the shoulders
- Shame/ Self-Hate affects our throat

I have a free mediation on YouTube you can find in the thank-you chapter that addresses these nine primary human emotions. It helps you bring up the negative emotions you have suppressed and assists you in clearing what you are ready to let go of. Emotional healing is like peeling layers off an onion. It takes some time to get to the core of the problem at hand. I recommend doing this meditation once a week for seven weeks. When you work on emotional healing, it has to surface to be released. You may have to refuel that emotion. When doing any sort of emotional healing, allow your body to feel the pain again but know it's coming up to be released so you can move on from it.

After my mom died, I was admittedly emotionally numb. I truly never cried it out, which scared me. My mom just died; how could I feel so emotion-less? I was such a mommy's girl. I cried every day from separation anxiety when she dropped me off at school until I reached second grade. What is going on? Well, I buried my grief so deep that I developed chronic pneumonia that lasted over a year. Every time it went away, it would come back a few months later. Grief affects lungs. Luckily, I was working with my naturopath, Jennifer, on my lungs. She told me about the correlation between grief and lung issues. We worked on the correlating emotion while supporting lung health, and I haven't had pneumonia since.

While writing this book I developed a severe kidney infection that came on out of nowhere. I'm talking level twelve out of ten pain that landed me in the emergency room at 4:00 a.m. I was stressed and feeling overwhelmed with the to-do list for my business and nonprofit. My life was rapidly changing, and I wasn't feeling very in control. Coincidently, the kidneys are affected by fear: fear of the unknown, fear of change. No wonder this was the area of my body that went down during this overwhelming time.

Was there a large emotional stressor that came up sometime within the year before you were diagnosed with cancer? What was happening in your life the year before you had cancer? If something comes up for you, I invite you to write an open letter to that pain, tragedy, or experience. Tell it how much you hated it, how it affected your life, and how awful it was to go through. Then tell it, "By releasing you, I set myself free." Next, write how much you learned from that experience, thank it for its lesson, and destroy that piece of paper. Rip it up, burn it, shred it – whatever makes you feel better. You won't forget what happened, but it will no longer have a hold over you, which sets your spirit free from that experience.

"True healing is integrated; treatment is specific, separate."
– Dr. Robert Morse

Chapter 8:

I HAVE A CLEAR PATH TO SUCCESS IN KEEPING MY BODY WELL

"Visualize your most beautiful and healthy self,
then start showing up as her."
– Unknown

I f you're feeling overwhelmed from everything you've learned so far, don't worry. I'm about to give you an eight-week guide to creating your new anti-cancer lifestyle. It is said that it takes twenty-one days to start a new habit. To assure your success, I will add an extra month to solidify these changes for long-lasting success. I know eight weeks may seem like a long time, but I want success and results for you. If you tried to change three different aspects of your life in twenty-one days, I would have failed you. I want life-changing results for you, not three weeks of making some healthy changes and then going back to old ways. Small, simple changes over time lead to big results. I made this plan so you can do it with ease and grace, not in a stressed and overwhelmed state.

The first month will focus on simple changes to get your diet on point, followed by lifestyle changes, and daily detox habits.

"When you feel like quitting, remember why you started!"

– Unknown

Week 1

- Visualize your most beautiful and healthy self every single day before you get out of bed. Visualize and journal how you want to look, feel, and live. What is your ideal healthy lifestyle? Journal what you want your daily routine to look like. Reflect to this once a day for the next three months.

- Reflect on any possible cancer-causing factors in your life. What key factors will you make a priority to change during this three-month journey?

- Drink half of your body weight in ounces of water a day (e.g., 200 pounds = 100 ounces of water).

- Start every morning with one of the simple fruit/veggie smoothies in the back of this book. The water you add to your smoothie can count toward your daily ounces.

Notes

Week 2

- Identify the major stressors in your life and come up with a list of creative solutions. Channel your belief system and know that one of these solutions will work out for you. Life is constant ebbs and flows. There are always good times and bad. If there is a chronic stressor in your life, let's work together to nix it before it becomes a health issue.

- Monitor the eighty/twenty rule of thumb: Eighty percent of your daily diet will be healthy fruits, vegetables, grains, and proteins; twenty percent will be processed food, chips, fried food, caffeine, dairy, sugar, and desserts. The closer to 100 percent you get, the better. I promise you that eating healthier over time will naturally cut cravings for bad foods. Your taste buds, and good gut bacteria, will change, leaving you with fewer cravings. The longer you eat a healthy diet, the easier it gets, and it gets harder to go back to old ways. You will no longer want the processed foods you once loved, and oftentimes if you cave and give it another go, you might feel lousy or sick. A healthy body will tell you what it doesn't want.

Notes

Week 3

- This week, work on proper food combining and eating lighter to heavier throughout the day:
  - Fruits in the morning
  - Fruits always eaten alone or with raw vegetables
  - Starches and vegetables
  - Protein and vegetables
  - Avoiding protein and starches at the same meal
  - These rules come pretty naturally when eating plant-based. If you choose to eat meat or fish here re two example meals.
  - Fish over a bed of sautéed greens; chicken with broccoli
- Try adding a probiotic supplement to your morning regimen until the end of this plan. A daily probiotic will help balance your gut while making changes in your diet.

Notes

Week 4

- Work toward getting the eighty/twenty rule closer to 100 percent clean eating.
- Your 100 percent clean diet should be eighty percent fruits and vegetables and twenty percent protein, carbohydrates, starches, and fats.
- This is a lifestyle, don't get discouraged if you fall off track. Consistency is the goal. Cheat meals that make you feel good here and there might be part of helping you sustain this goal.
- Work on cutting back dairy and meat, leaving them for only one meal of the day.
- If you choose to continue with meat and dairy, choose organic and hormone-free if possible.

"Do something today that your future self will thank you for."

– Unknown

Notes

Week 5

- This week, work on swapping your most used self-care products for healthier alternatives.
- E.g.: replacing artificially scented body lotion with a natural alternative or coconut oil, swapping your skin-care routine for a more natural alternative, replacing your perfume with a naturally scented one or essential oil blend.

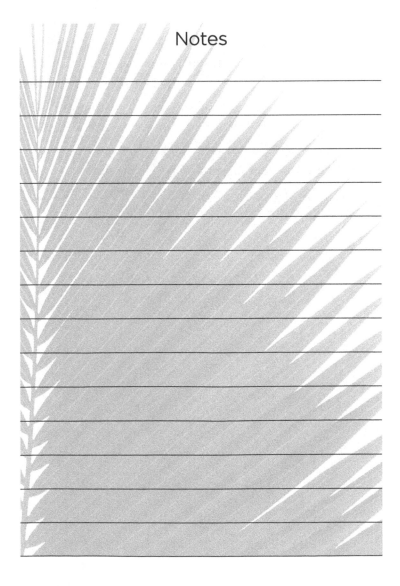

Notes

Week 6

- This week, we will create a healthier living environment.
- Replace the candles and air fresheners around the house with a clean-burning candle (e.g.: soy or beeswax-based).
- I like to create a room spray by buying a spray bottle of rose water and adding essential oils to it.
- Look into getting an air filter for the most-used room of the house.
- Replace toxic laundry detergent with a natural alternative.
- Switch the hand soaps in your house with a natural alternative that is free of perfume and dyes.
- Unplug the Wi-Fi router before bed.

Notes

Week 7

- This week, we will incorporate detox strategies.
- Get a good sweat at least one to three times a week. I have a $100 personal steam sauna that I bought from Amazon, and it is the greatest thing ever. I use it for about fifteen minutes a few times a week. Does your gym have a sauna? You could use that. If not either of these, a hot bath with Epsom or magnesium flakes will do the trick, I promise.
- Oil pull for five minutes a day. Oil pulling is when you swish oil around in your mouth which helps to draw impurities from the mouth and back of the throat. I use coconut oil and do this for five to ten minutes before brushing my teeth. It is so good to do if you have any congestion in your head or back of the throat. It helps to clear that area.
- Do a self-massage all over for good blood flow and lymphatic system support a few times a week.
- Do a foot massage every night this week. It will hit all the reflexology points on your feet which helps to unblock stagnant energy for the organs according to Chinese medicine.
- Do a stomach massage before bed or when you wake up in the morning for good digestion and to keep things moving. Massage in a clockwise, circular motion.
- Add an herbal tea to your daily regimen. My favorites are peppermint or fennel for good digestion, chamomile for bedtime relaxation, lemon balm for antibacterial properties, and raspberry leaf for anything related to the female reproductive system.

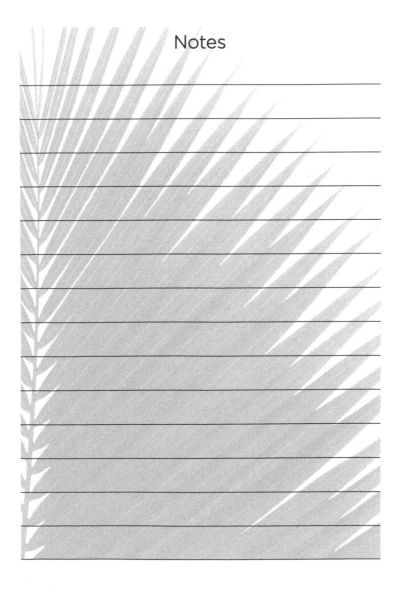

Notes

Week 8

- This week, we will create a movement regimen and tie up loose ends.
- Create a two-minute stretching routine that you will do when you wake up in the morning and before you go to bed.
- What is your favorite form of exercise? Create an exercise routine you will stick to.
- Go over the previous tasks and access where you have fallen behind. Work on incorporating those into your lifestyle.

Download a printable eight weeks to Keeping Well chart on my website in the back of this book.

"If you don't program yourself,
your environment will."
– Unknown

Notes

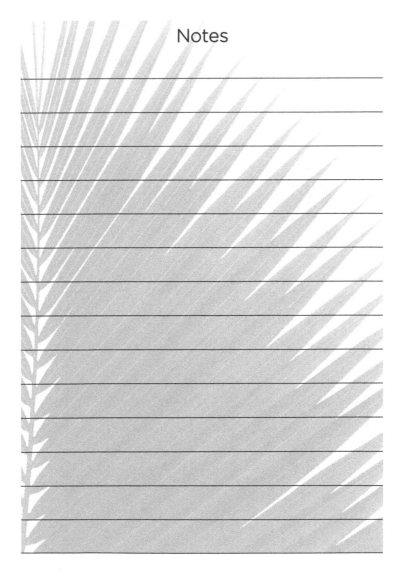

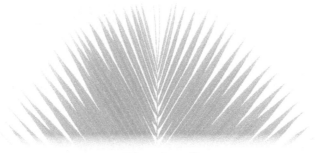

Chapter 9:

I WILL LIVE MY LIFE
WITH EASE AND GRACE

L ife is a constant motion of natural ebbs and flows. Nothing is stationary; everything is constantly changing. No bad thing ever lasts. My mom would always tell me, "This too shall pass." Any obstacle you face toward keeping well will always reach a breakthrough.

Self-doubt will stop you more than any other force is capable of. You can achieve anything if you get over your own hurdles first, self-doubt almost stopped me from writing this book. I had so many doubtful thoughts popping up: Who am I to write about cancer? I'm not a doctor; I've never had cancer. I have breast implants, which are not health-promoting. Will people even take me seriously? You know what I finally thought? This book has been in the making in my head for the past nine years, and if I don't write it:

1. It would haunt me until I did
2. It would be doing a huge disservice to my ideal reader, who is looking for ways to get healthy after cancer and I don't take that lightly.

I wrote this book as if I could travel back in time and hand it to my mom after her first go with cancer. I know for a fact my mom would have been so open to the information in here, and if one other person reading this is too, then I would be awful not write this book because I didn't feel good enough.

If you're thinking it will be too hard to break old habits or start a new anti-cancer lifestyle, it will be – at least until you get over your own stuff that is stopping you from wanting it bad enough. If you're reading this book to get healthy, then hold your ideal vision of what healthy looks like in your head and want it bad enough that you will commit yourself to it no matter what.

That's what I did for this book. I wrote it, and I put it out there for everyone to see, read, and review. Let me tell you, it was not easy. There was a mini breakdown over the fear of backlash for having breast implants and simultaneously writing about toxin exposure. Trust me, I get the hypocrisy, but I realized it was a gift. It helped me correlate my message of not worrying about being perfect, staying on track, and accessing your own risk management. This whole book is about the process, not perfection.

You Have to Assess Your Risk Management

Your mental health and feeling good about your body is an important part of healing. That is part of the holistic approach to keeping well. I know that if I removed my breast implants today for health reasons, the emotional and mental backlash might outweigh the potential physical harm they are doing to my body. I assessed my risk, and I choose my outcome based on my knowledge at this time.

You have to assess your own risk management. There are plenty of unhealthy things in this world, and you would go crazy if you were obsessed about doing everything to absolute health perfection. Reducing stress and enjoying life is key in reducing the risk of cancer. So if you slip up on your Keeping Well lifestyle, don't stress; just get back on track.

Mitigation Techniques to Enjoy Life to The Fullest and Reverse the Damage

I am all about living in balance and not feeling guilty when you want to have a drink or a feel-good meal with friends. I want you to maintain results without feeling restricted. Living in deprivation or guilt over a cupcake or margarita is a negative emotion. Negative emotions lower our body's energy and immune system, so why not thoroughly enjoy them on occasion when you know how to reverse the damage? Guiltlessly have fun but learn how to heal from a night out with these mitigation techniques.

After having an unhealthy meal that leaves you feeling not so great:

- Have some ginger, peppermint, or fennel tea.
- Take a digestive enzyme before and after. Sunfood Digestive Enzymes is one I have used. There are also papaya chewable enzymes like the Country Life Tropical Papaya. These help promote nutrient absorption and digestive discomforts.
- Have a few fennel seeds and chew them like mints.
- Lie on your left-hand side when you go to sleep that night; this is the side you want to sleep on for optimal digestion.

After having an alcoholic drink:

- Take activated charcoal first thing in the morning or before bed. This will help soak up the toxins from drinking; however, it will also soak up other things, so make sure to take it two hours before taking the following recommendations.
- Take a probiotic before and the morning after drinking to replenish healthy gut bacteria.
- Have coconut water the following day for dehydration and electrolyte replenishment. It is the world's purest liquid next to water.
- Add trace mineral drops to your water or coconut water to also boost electrolyte and healthy cell salt replenishment
- Make a super hydrating fruit smoothie with water or coconut water and add a few tablespoons of hemp seeds, which are super nutrient-rich in healthy fats and vitamins.
- Have a cooling and anti-inflammatory green juice like cucumber juice.
- Apply a drop of peppermint essential oil to the back of your neck to help with feeling dizzy.

According to the CDC, the less alcohol you drink, the lower your risk for cancer. Drinking alcohol raises your risk of getting six kinds of cancer:

- Mouth and throat
- Voice box (larynx)
- Esophagus
- Colon and rectum
- Liver
- Breast (in women)[18]

Alcohol makes the body acidic, which creates inflammation and heat. We want a nice cool and neutral body that is in homeostasis and not constant active repair mode. Constant inflammation damages healthy tissues. Cancer is damaged cells. Just keep this in mind when doing anything damaging to the body, and you will notice how your choices improve.

As humans we always make decisions based on our current level of awareness. This book is simply about bringing awareness to the things that are keeping our body unhealthy so that the new decisions you make are from a healthier perspective.

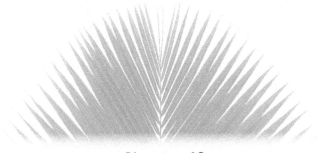

Chapter 10:

I AM DEDICATED TO HEALING MY BODY AND KEEPING WELL BECAUSE I AM WORTHY OF HAVING A PERFECTLY HEALTHY BODY AND FEELING GREAT

"Be strong. You never know who you are inspiring."
– Unknown

I f you haven't noticed, each chapter title is a healing affirmation you can say to yourself daily to anchor in the mind-body healing connection. Repeat these affirmations for the next twenty-one days. I encourage you to handwrite these out to create a deeper connection in your own way.

- I am choosing to remain cancer-free.
- I am open to receiving guidance.
- I am keeping my body well by learning from and listening to it.
- I understand how my body works, so I know how to heal it.
- I know my body has the ability to heal itself and I am assisting it in every way.
- I create a healthy environment all around me.
- I welcome all emotions to be healed.
- I have a clear path to success in keeping my body well.
- I will live my life with ease and grace.
- I am dedicated to healing my body and keeping well because I am worthy of having a perfectly healthy body and feeling great.

I hope that by integrating the Keeping Well process from this book, you know what it is like to feel true health. Most people do not know what it is like to feel true health. To feel like a fully healthy human being is to feel full of energy, connected to all living things, living in balance, and having a healthy functioning body to experience all of this.

"Most people have no idea how good their body is designed to feel."
– Kevin Trudeau

Stay on the healing path. Small changes over time create a huge compounded change. It can be for the better or the worse. The choice is up to you, but in ten more years, you will be down one of those roads no matter what. It all depends on the daily choices you make. I hope this book has helped you navigate the path a little better. I also hope this book gives you inspiration to dive deeper into learning about self-healing techniques that can change your life and all others around you who learn from your example.

Stay encouraged and inspired to be the healthiest, most beautiful version of yourself.

"I hope you love yourself enough to recognize the things you don't like about your life, and I hope you have the courage to change them."
– Unknown

ACKNOWLEDGMENTS

Thank you to Angela Lauria and The Author Incubator's team, as well as to David Hancock and the Morgan James Publishing team for helping me bring this book to print.

THANK YOU

I have left many gifts for you throughout this book that you can download from the link below. They include download-able charts for you to keep your anti-cancer journey on track, an affirmation list, an emotional healing meditation, and recom-mended products. I also have included a bonus video, *Keeping Well after Cancer: 7 Pillars to Optimal Health*. Don't forget to share it with a friend whom you think would benefit. You can find all of these at www.BrittanyWisniewski.com/Keepingwell

If you want to dive deeper and work with me personally, please check out my website www.BrittanyWisniewski.com

Additionally, I have created a Facebook group for anyone looking for support and encouragement while keeping well after cancer. You can find it at https://www.facebook.com/groups/2741713589288424/

Find your Keeping Well support system by sharing your journey to wellness on Instagram and other social media platforms by using the hashtag #keepingwell. Follow me on Instagram at @BrittanyNWisniewski for daily updates.

ABOUT THE AUTHOR

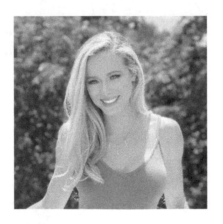

Brittany Wisniewski is a detoxification specialist who helps cancer survivors create a sustainable healthy lifestyle to do their best to remain in remission. Her expertise is in preventative care using proper nutrition, detox strategies, and emotional wellbeing. Brittany channeled the grief of losing her mom to breast cancer into learning everything she could about anti-cancer wellness.

Brittany has been in the natural health and wellness field for a decade. She has helped countless clients detoxify their bodies to reach optimal health and is an expert in organic skin care and detoxification.

Brittany became a regenerative detoxification specialist through the International School of Detoxification in 2017. She earned a certification in plant-based nutrition from eCornell. She is an avid learner and currently studying traditional naturopathy at New Eden School of Natural Health.

She now combines her many areas of expertise in the natural health arena to assist cancer survivors in restoring their health after cancer. She provides private and group trainings that help her clients remove disease causing factors in their life and create a sustainable anti-cancer lifestyle to remain in remission.

Brittany believes everyone deserves optimal health, which established her passion project in 2019 – Keep Well, a 501(c)(3) non-profit whose mission is to fund holistic care for cancer patients.

Brittany was born and raised in Baltimore, Maryland, where she still resides in her palm tree filled home.

ENDNOTES

1   https://www.ncbi.nlm.nih.gov/pmc/articles/
    PMC2515569/

2   Sloan EK, Priceman SJ, Cox BF, et al. The sympathetic
    nervous system induces a metastatic switch in primary
    breast cancer. Cancer Research 2010;70(18):7042–52.
    [PubMed Abstract]

3   https://www.ewg.org/skindeep/2004/06/15/exposures-add-
    up-survey-results/

4   https://www.cdc.gov/biomonitoring/Phthalates_FactSheet.
    html

5   https://www.ncbi.nlm.nih.gov/pmc/articles/
    PMC4902544/

6   https://www.breastcancer.org/risk/factors/low_vit_d/

7   https://www.ncbi.nlm.nih.gov/pmc/articles/
    PMC5802611/

8   https://www.fda.gov/news-events/fda-voices-perspec-
    tives-fda-leadership-and-experts/shedding-new-light-sun-
    screen-absorption#2

9   https://www.researchgate.net/publication/261516659_
    Chronic_High-Fat_Diet_Impairs_Collecting_Lymphatic_
    Vessel_Function_in_Mice

10 https://www.ncbi.nlm.nih.gov/pmc/articles/
    PMC3945755/

11 https://scripps.ucsd.edu/news/study-finds-toxic-pollutants-
    fish-across-worlds-oceans/
    https://www.who.int/features/qa/cancer-red-meat/en/

12 https://www.cancer.org/cancer/cancer-causes/recombi-
    nant-bovine-growth-hormone.html

13 https://www.ewg.org/research/rethinking-carcinogens/hali-
    fax-project-complete-vs-partial-carcinogens

14 https://www.ewg.org/research/chromium-six-found-in-us-
    tap-water/

15 https://www.endocrine.org/news-room/current-press-re-
    leases/exposure-to-bpa-substitute-bps-multiplies-breast-
    cancer-cells

16 https://www.ncbi.nlm.nih.gov/pubmed/29913098/

17 https://www.ncbi.nlm.nih.gov/pubmed/30343375/

18 https://www.cdc.gov/cancer/alcohol/index.htm

CPSIA information can be obtained
at www.ICGtesting.com
Printed in the USA
JSHW010715121120
9521JS00004B/181